MDSAP

Vol.4 of 5 Japan

For All

(Employees & Employers)

Second Edition:

Online Certification

www.silosa.ca

Jahangir Asadi

Vancouver, BC CANADA

I0047005

Copyright © 2022 by **SILOSA** Consulting Group Inc.

All rights reserved. No part of this publication may be reproduced, distributed or transmitted in any form or by any means, including photocopying, recording, or other electronic or mechanical methods, without the prior written permission of the publisher, except in the case of brief quotations embodied in critical reviews and certain other noncommercial uses permitted by copyright law. For permission requests, write to the publisher, addressed "Attention: Permissions Coordinator," at the address below.

Published by: Silosa Consulting Group Inc.
Vancouver, BC **CANADA**
Email: Info@Silosa.ca
www.silosa.ca

Ordering Information:
Quantity sales. Special discounts are available on quantity purchases by universities, schools, corporations, associations, and others. For details, contact the "Sales Department" at the above mentioned email address.

MDSAP Vol.1-5 (for all employees and employers)/J.Asadi—2nd ed.

ISBN	Vol	Country	Format
978-1-990451-55-3	Vol.1	Australia	Paperback
978-1-990451-56-0	Vol.2	Brazil	Paperback
978-1-990451-57-7	Vol.3	Canada	Paperback
978-1-990451-58-4	Vol.4	Japan	Paperback
978-1-990451-59-1	Vol.5	USA	Paperback

Contents

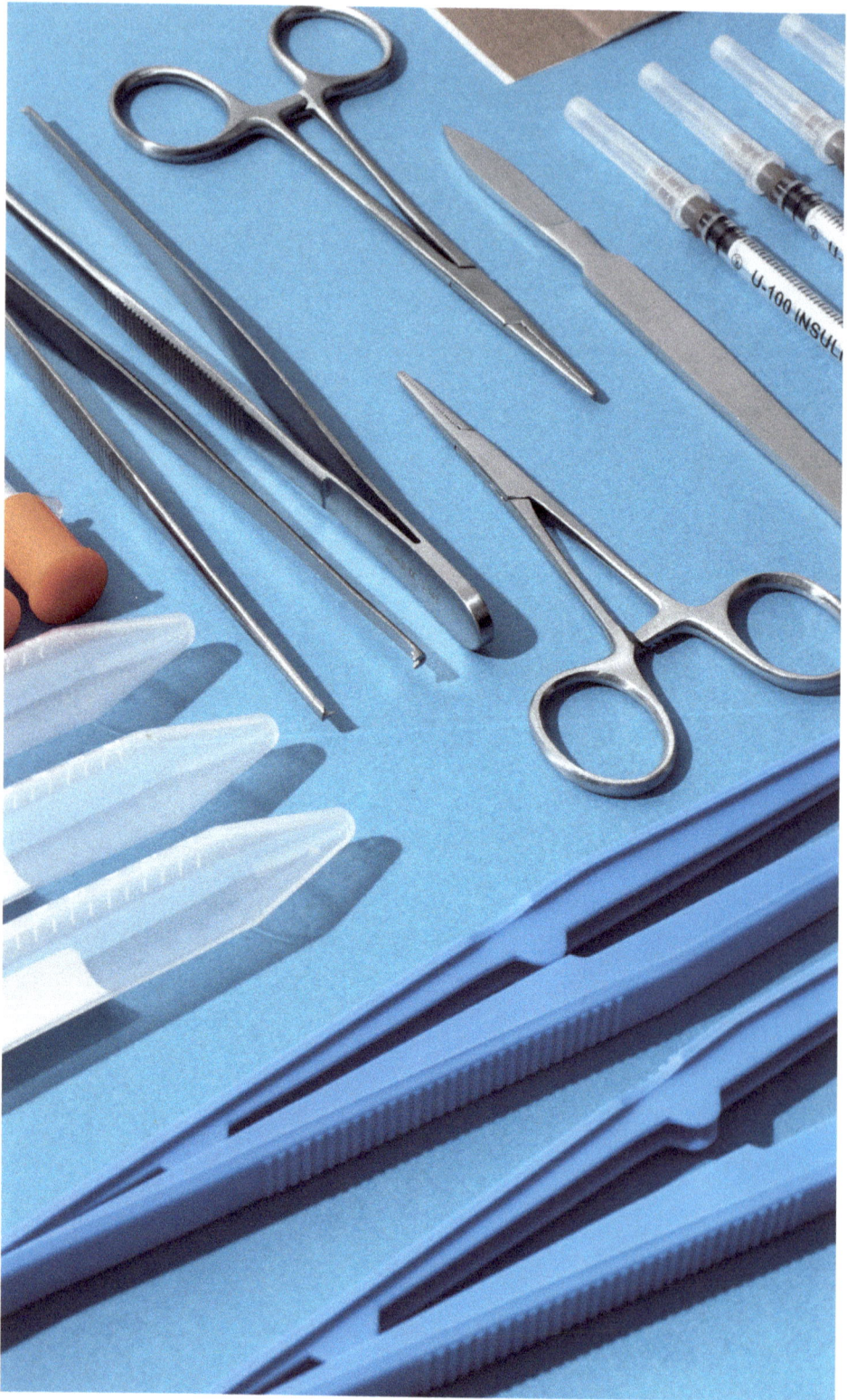

This book is dedicated to my first manager,

Mir Ahmad Sadat,

a Distinguished man of ISIRI, who has been my supporter and has encouraged me greatly and believed genuinely in my ability with honesty and self-confidence.

Every possible effort has been made to ensure that the information contained in this book is accurate at the time of going to press, and the publishers and the author cannot accept responsibility for any errors or omissions, however caused. No responsibility for loss or damage occasioned to any person acting, or refraining from action, as a result of the material in this publication can be accepted by the publisher and/or the author.

SILOSA Consulting Group (SCG)

Silosa Consulting Group (SCG) was established to provide outstanding consulting services of management system standards to individuals, groups, companies, and organizations all over the globe.

SCG is publishing an "EASY ISO" book series related to International Management System Standards to increase public knowledge in implementing these systems over their organizations.

SCG book publishing services and distribution services are connected to over 39,000 booksellers worldwide, including Apple, Amazon, Barnes & Noble, Indigo, Google Play Books, and many more. We focus on quality, environmental, food safety and other management system standards.

SCG has enough experiences to help create new and effective programmes in different countries all over the world. For more detail, visit our
website : http://silosa.ca and/or   send your enquiery to the following email:

info@silosa.ca

About ISO

The International Organization for Standardization is an independent, non-governmental organization, the members of which are the standards organizations of the 165 member countries. It is the world's largest developer of voluntary international standards and it facilitates world trade by providing common standards among nations. More than twenty thousand standards have been set, covering everything from manufactured products and technology to food safety, agriculture, and healthcare.

Use of the standards aids in the creation of products and services that are safe, reliable, and of good quality. The standards help businesses increase productivity while minimizing errors and waste. By enabling products from different markets to be directly compared, they facilitate companies in entering new markets and assist in the development of global trade on a fair basis. The standards also serve to safeguard consumers and the end-users of products and services, ensuring that certified products conform to the minimum standards set internationally.

2nd Edition

History

The organization began in the 1920s as the International Federation of the National Standardizing Associations (ISA). It was suspended in 1942 during World War II, but after the war ISA was approached by the recently formed United Nations Standards Coordinating Committee (UNSCC) with a proposal to form a new global standards body. In October 1946, ISA and UNSCC delegates from 25 countries met in London and agreed to join forces to create the new International Organization for Standardization. The new organization officially began operations in February 1947.

More information can be obtained :

www.ISO.org

Geneva, Switzerlan (Headquarter of ISO)

CHAPTER 2

MDSAP

MDSAP The Medical Device Single Audit Program is the single audit program that covers the regulations of Australia, Brazil, Canada, Japan and USA. These regulations use the MDSAP to verify compliance to the quality systems of their national regulations and ISO 13485. The intention of the Medical Device Single Audit Program (MDSAP) is to allow competent auditors from MDSAP recognized Auditing Organizations (AOs) to conduct a single audit of a medical device organization's quality management system that will satisfy the requirements of the medical device regulatory authorities participating in the MDSAP program.
Audits performed under the MDSAP program will be process based, focusing on several defined processes, a defined method for linking those processes, and built on a foundation of requirements for risk management.

ISO 13485 MDSAP are two different programs with similar requirements but they do not duplicate each other.
MDSAP has the more stringent requirements of the two and companies that are already certified to ISO 13485 will see an increase in the number of audit days once they seek certification to MDSAP. The design of the Medical Device Single Audit Program (MDSAP) audit process is to ensure a single audit will provide efficient yet thorough coverage of regulatory requirements.
These requirements include; Medical devices – Quality management systems – Requirements for regulatory purposes (ISO 13485:2016), the Quality Management System requirements of the Conformity Assessment Procedures of the Australian Therapeutic

Goods (Medical Devices) Regulations (TG(MD)R Sch3), the Bra-
zilian Good Manufacturing Practices (RDC ANVISA 16/2013),
the Japanese Ordinance on Standards for Manufacturing Control
and Quality Control of Medical Devices and In Vitro Diagnostic
Reagents (MHLW Ministerial Ordinance No. 169), the Quality System Regulation (21 CFR Part 820), and specific requirements of
the medical device regulatory authorities participating in the MD-
SAP program.

What is the meaning of ISO 13485 certified?

ISO certification is a seal of approval from a third party body that a
company runs to one of the international standards developed and
published by the International Organization for Standardization
(ISO). ... ISO 13485 helps put your customers first.

Is ISO 13485 certification worth it?

ISO 13485 is important to designers, manufacturers, and distribu-
tors of medical devices. In addition, suppliers and service provid-
ers can enhance an organization's marketability as more and more
manufacturers require certification in order to do business with a
vendor.

MDSAP AUDIT:

The design and development of the MDSAP audit sequence allows
a logical, focused and efficient conduct of an audit. The MDSAP
audit sequence follows a process approach and has four primary
processes - Management process, Measurement, Analysis and Improvement process, Design and Development process and a Production and Service Controls process with links to the supporting
process for Purchasing.

The definition of each process includes a purpose and an outcome
that are indicators of process performance. Each participating Regulatory Authority expects that risk management to be the foundation for the five processes that are the requirements of a quality
management system for medical device organizations.

The MDSAP audit process has two additional supporting processes: Device Marketing Authorization and Facility Registration and Medical Device Adverse Events and Advisory Notices Reporting. These processes are necessary to fulfill specific requirements of the participating MDSAP regulatory authorities.

Regulatory Requirements

Country	Regulatory	MDSAP
Australia	Conformity Assessment Procedures of the Australian Therapeutic Goods (Medical Devices) Regulations (TG(MD)R Sch3)	Vo.1
Brazil	The Brazilian Good Manufacturing Practices (RDC ANVISA 2013/16)	Vol.2
Canada	Medical Devices Regulations SOR/282-98 and specific requirements of the medical device regulatory authorities	Vol.3
Japan	The Japanese Ordinance on Standards for Manufacturing Control and Quality Control of Medical Devices and In Vitro Diagnostic Reagents (MHLW Ministerial Ordinance No. 169),	Vol.4
USA	FDA Quality System Regulation (21 CFR Part 820)	Vol.5

United States of America   Japan   Canada   Brazil   Australia

Definitions

ISO 13485 specifies requirements for a quality management system where an organization needs to demonstrate its ability to provide medical devices and related services that consistently meet customer and applicable regulatory requirements. Such organizations can be involved in one or more stages of the life-cycle, including design and development, production, storage and distribution, installation, or servicing of a medical device and design and development or provision of associated activities (e.g. technical support). ISO 13485 can also be used by suppliers or external parties that provide product, including quality management system-related services to such organizations.

Scope of Certificate: The scope of the ISO certificate depends on how your Organization would like to have keeping in view of future. Some want to be specific by listing the products; some to be general covering the broad category of products. Here are some examples:

1. Design, development assemble, manufacture, distribute and service of life science instruments

2. Design, assemble/manufacture, sales & service of medical instruments used in cardiology including ECG Recorders, Bedside monitors

3. Design, development, manufacture, distribute and repair of medical device instruments intended to use in genetic analysis such as DNA Amplifiers, Genetic Analyzers, etc.

Distributer

Natural or legal person in the supply chain who, on his own behalf, furthers the availability of a medical device to the end user

Importer

natural or legal person in the supply chain who is the first in a supply chain to make a medical device,

manufactured in another country or jurisdiction, available in the country or jurisdiction where it is to

be marketed

Manufacturer

natural or legal person with responsibility for design and/or manufacture of a medical device with the

intention of making the medical device available for use, under his name; whether or not such a medical

device is designed and/or manufactured by that person himself or on his behalf by another person(s)

Device The term "device" is used throughout the MDSAP processes. For the purpose of applying the MDSAP processes, and to accommodate nuances in the regulatory systems of the participating Regulatory Authorities, the use of the term "device" is to refer to any product that is capable of functioning as a medical device, whether or not it is packaged, labeled, or sterilized.

Supplier: Organization or individual that enters into an agreement with the acquirer or integrator for the supply of a product or service.

We can categorized the suppliers to:
• Critical Supplier
• Non-critical supplier

A purchased or otherwise obtained "product" or "service" is an outsourced product or service. In addition, a "supplier" is anyone that is independent from the medical device organization's quality management system. This includes a supplier that may be part of the same corporation as the medical device organization but operates under a separate quality management system from the audited medical device organization.

Critical Suppliers:

For the purposes of MDSAP, "critical suppliers" include, but are not limited to;

• Those entities that supply the organization with finished devices, i.e. a device, or accessory to any device, that is suitable for use or capable of functioning, whether or not it is packaged, labeled, or sterilized;
• Suppliers of products, including services, that impact design outputs that are essential for the proper functioning of the device; and
• Suppliers of products and services that require process validation.

Not all MDSAP participating regulatory authorities require, or make use of, certification documents that relate to a medical device organization's QMS. The terms "certification" and "recertification" appear within this volumes to maintain consistency with the terminology used within ISO/IEC 17021-1:2015 Conformity assessment – Requirements for bodies providing audit and certification of management systems.

MDSAP Audit

The Medical Device Single Audit Program is based on a three (3) year audit cycle. The Initial Audit, also referred to as the "Initial Certification Audit" is a complete audit of a medical device organization's quality management system (QMS) consisting of:

Stage 1 Audit (17021-1:2015 – Cl 9.3.1.2)

Stage 2 Audit (17021-1:2015 – Cl 9.3.1.3)

The initial Audit is followed by a partial Surveillance Audit (17021-1:2015 – Cl 9.6.2.2) in each of the following two (2) years and a complete Re-audit, also referred to as a "Recertification Audit" (17021-1:2015 – Cl 9.6.3.2) in the third (3rd) year. A recertification audit may also include a Stage 1 audit if there have been significant changes to the QMS that have not been otherwise adequately assessed.

Initial Certification Audit

Initial Certification audit consists of: Stage 1 & 2

Stage 1

Documentation review, evaluation of preparedness for Stage 2 audit, etc.

A Stage 1 audit shall be conducted in accordance with Clause 9.3.1.2 of ISO/IEC 17021-1:2015 and all applicable MDSAP Audit Process tasks and regulatory requirements.

From an MDSAP perspective, the primary purposes of a Stage 1 audit are (1) to determine if QMS documentation required by ISO 13485:2016 - Clauses 4.2.1 and other applicable MDSAP documentation requirements have been adequately defined, and documented; (2) to assess the medical device organization's preparedness for a Stage 2 audit; (3) to provide a focus for planning a Stage 2 audit; and, (4) to collect information regarding the scope of the quality management system and other aspects of the medical device organization.

Portions of a Stage 1 audit (e.g. documentation review) may be performed at a site other than the site(s) of the medical device organization seeking initial certification.

The outcome of the Stage 1 audit will assist the MDSAP recognized Auditing Organization in its determination of the readiness of the medical device organization to undergo a Stage 2 audit. The Au-

diting Organization shall determine how best to accomplish tasks of Stage 1 and Stage 2 with regards to off-site documentation and record review and on-site verifications. Hence portions of a Stage 1 audit (e.g. documentation review) may be performed at a site other than the site(s) of the medical device organization seeking initial certification. In practice it is intended that the Auditing Organization may combine elements of Stage 1 and Stage 2 to allow for a single on-site visit for the initial audit or re-audit of the medical device organization.

Stage 2

Evaluation of QMS Implementation and Effectiveness

A Stage 2 audit shall be conducted in accordance with Clause 9.3.1.3 of ISO/IEC 17021-1:2015 and using all applicable MDSAP Audit Process tasks.

The purpose of a Stage 2 audit is to determine if all applicable requirements of ISO 13485:2016 and the relevant regulatory requirements from participating regulatory authorities have been implemented. Stage 2 audit objectives shall specifically include an evaluation of:

- The effectiveness of the medical device organization's QMS incorporating the applicable regulatory requirements;
- Product/process related technologies (e.g. injection molding, sterilization);
- Adequate product technical documentation in relation to relevant regulatory requirements; and,
- The medical device organization's ability to comply with these requirements.

Surveillance Audits

(1st and 2nd Surveillance Audits):

A Surveillance Audit shall be conducted in accordance with Clause 9.6.2.2 of ISO/IEC 17021-1:2015 and clause 9.6.2 of IMDRF/MDSAP WG/N3:2016 and using applicable MDSAP Audit Process tasks. The purpose of a series of surveillance audits is to assure that all applicable requirements of ISO 13485:2016 and the relevant regulatory requirements from participating regulatory authorities are audited during the cycle of a three year audit program for the medical device organization. Surveillance audit objectives during the audit cycle shall specifically include evaluation of:

- The effectiveness of the medical device organization's QMS incorporating the applicable regulatory requirements.
- The medical device organization's ability to comply with these requirements; and
- New or changed product/process related technologies; and,
- New or amended product technical documentation in relation to relevant regulatory requirements.

In addition, surveillance audits shall include a review of issues related to medical device safety and effectiveness since the last audit such as complaints, problem reports, vigilance reports, and recalls/ field corrections/advisory notices.

Re-audit (Recertification Audits)

A Re-audit (Recertification Audit) shall be conducted in accordance with Clause 9.6.3 of ISO/IEC 17021-1:2015 and using all applicable MDSAP Audit Process tasks. The purpose of a re-audit is

All Rights Reserved by:
Silosa Consulting Group Inc.

Sample Q

as a P

ISO 13
MD

Your Company
Quality Plan

Your Company
Organizational Chart

You
Produc

Vision

Mi

ity Manual

STER

5:2016

AP

Procedural

Flowchart

Refereing to all

QMS procedures

and

Work Instructions

dical

ervices

Value

to confirm the continued relevance, applicability and suitability of the medical device organization's QMS (as a whole), to satisfy all applicable requirements of ISO 13485:2016 and the relevant regulatory requirements from participating regulatory authorities, with respect to the scope of certification. Recertification audit objectives shall specifically include evaluation of:

- the effectiveness of the medical device organization's QMS incorporating the applicable regulatory requirements
- product/process related technologies (e.g. injection molding, sterilization)
- adequate product technical documentation in relation to relevant regulatory requirements
- the medical device organization's continued fulfillment of these requirements.

United States of America — Japan — Canada — Brazil — Australia

Audits Conducted by Regulatory Authorities

Audits may also be conducted by MDSAP participating regulatory authorities at any time and for a range of reasons including (1) "For Cause" due to information obtained by the regulatory authority, (2) as follow up to the findings of a previous audit, and (3) to confirm the effective implementation of MDSAP requirements by MDSAP recognized auditing organizations.

The purpose of audits conducted by regulatory authorities is to ensure appropriate oversight of a recognized MDSAP Auditing Organization's audit activities, as an alternative means of assessing medical device organizations that have been identified as undertaking high risk manufacturing processes and have not been adequately audited, where sufficient detail regarding audited processes has not been included in an audit report, or where there is a history of low compliance with QMS or regulatory requirements.

MDSAP
ISO 13485 Requirements &

JAPAN
MAP

Management

The intent of the Management Process is to provide adequate resources for device design, manufacturing, quality assurance, distribution, installation, and servicing activities; to assure the quality management system is functioning properly and effectively; and to monitor the quality management system and make necessary adjustments. A quality management system that has been implemented effectively and is monitored to identify and address existing and potential problems is more likely to produce medical devices that function as intended.

The management representative is responsible for ensuring that the requirements of the quality management system have been effectively defined, documented, implemented, and maintained. Prior to the audit of a process, it may be helpful to interview the management representative (or designee) to obtain an overview of the process and a feel for management's knowledge and understanding of the process.

Clause and Regulation:
ISO 13485:2016: 4.1.1, 4.1.2, 4.1.3, 4.2.2, 4.1.4, 5.4.2;
MHLW/PMDA: MHLW MO169: 5, 7, 14;
MHLW/PMDA: MHLW MO169: 16, 18, 19, 20
MHLW/PMDA: MHLW MO169: 10, 15, 16, 21, 22, 23, 26

Japan

Confirm that Quality Management System documentation and re-cords in relation to a device are retained for the following periods (5 years for training records and documentation). [MHLW MO169: 8.4, 9.3, 67, 68]. (1) 15 years for 'specially designated maintenance control required medical devices' [or one year plus the shelf life for products when the shelf life or the expiry date (hereinafter simply referred to as the "shelf life") plus one year exceeds 15 years]. (2) 5 years for the products other than the 'specially designated mainte-nance control required medical devices' (or one year plus the shelf life for the products of which the shelf life plus one year exceeds 5 years).

Note: The 'specially designated maintenance control required medi-cal device' is defined as below in PMD Act 2.8:

A medical device designated by the Minister of Health, Labour and Welfare after hearing the opinion of the Pharmaceutical Affairs and Food Sanitation Council as those whose potential risk to the diagno-sis, treatment or prevention of disease is significant without proper control since this kind of equipment requires expert knowledge and skill in examination for maintenance and inspection, repair and oth-er management.

Device Marketing Authorization and Facility Registration

The Device Marketing Authorization and Facility Registration process may be audited as a linkage from the Management process and/or the Design and Development process.

ISO: ISO 13485:2016: 4.1.1, 4.2.1, 5.2, 7.2.1, 7.2.3
[PMD Act 23-2-3.1, 23-2-4]
[PMD Act 23-2-12]

Japan

"Marketing Authorization Holder" means a person who resides in Japan and is granted a license for marketing from a prefecture government [PMD Act 23-2.1].

Application or Notification for marketing

Class 2, class 3, and class 4 medical devices except for the ones specified by the requirement of PMD Act 23-2-23.1.

An" Application for Marketing Approval" shall be submitted to PMDA by the Marketing Authorization Holder to get authorization for marketing a medical device in Japan. [PMD Act 23-2-5.1]

An "Application for QMS Audit" shall also be submitted to PMDA by the Marketing Authorization Holder, when they do not have an effective QMS Certificate for the device. [PMD Act 23-2-5.6, 7]

Class 2 and class 3 medical devices which are specified by the requirement of PMD Act 23-2-23.1

An" Application for Marketing Certification" shall be submitted to a Registered Certification Body (RCB) by the Marketing Authorization Holder to get authorization for marketing a medical device in Japan. [PMD Act 23-2-23.1].

An "Application for QMS Audit" shall also be submitted to an RCB by the person, when the person does not have a valid QMS Certificate for the device. [PMD Act 23-2-23.3, 4].

Class 1 medical device

"Notification for Marketing" shall be submitted to PMDA by the Marketing Authorization Holder for marketing a class 1 device in Japan [PMD Act 23-2-12].

A class 1 medical device doesn't need any QMS Certificate for marketing.

Facility Registration (Registered Manufacturing Site)

A medical device manufacturing site which conducts one of the designated manufacturing processes listed below shall be registered:
- Main Designing
- Main assembly
- Sterilization
- Domestic storage before final release.

The site is called "Registered Manufacturing Site". It has to submit an application to PMDA for registration by itself [PMD Act 23-2-3.1, 23-2-4].

Any person who intends to market a medical device for business in Japan shall have a license for marketing granted by the prefectural government. This person is called a "Marketing Authorization Holder" (MAH) and shall reside in Japan [PMD Act 23-2.1]. The person has to submit an Application for Marketing Approval/Certification (class 2, 3 or 4 medical device) or a Notification for Marketing (class 1 medical device) to get marketing clearance for the medical device. No person shall market a medical device in Japan, unless the Marketing Authorization Holder of the device has been granted the marketing clearance [PMD Act 23-2-5.1, 23-2-23.1, 23-2-12].

A change to a medical device which is approved/certified by PMDA/a Registered Certification Body may require the Marketing Authorization Holder to submit a new application, a change application, or a change notification [PMD Act 23-2-5.1, 23-2-5.11, 23-2-5.12, 23-2-23.1, 23-2-23.6, 23-2-23.7].

Changes that require the application or the notification are those ones which directly impact the safety and efficacy of the device and/or the substantial identity of the fact approved during marketing approval / certification.

The Registered Manufacturing Site shall communicate with the Marketing Authorization Holder about the change when the Registered Manufacturing Site plans such changes, so that the Marketing Authorization Holder could take any necessary regulatory actions mentioned above [MHLW MO169; 29].

Examples of changes that may require an application or a notification include, but are not limited to, the following:
- Design
- Composition
- Raw material
- Sterilization method
- Manufacturing method
- Manufacturing site
- Patient or user safety features
- Operating Parameters or conditions for use
- Indication for use
- Shelf life
- Performance Specification.

Measurement, Analysis and Improvement

One of the most important activities in the quality management system is the identification of existing and potential causes of product and quality problems. Such causes must be identified so that appropriate and effective corrective or preventive actions can take place. These activities are carried out under the Measurement, Analysis and Improvement process.

Clause and Regulation
ISO: ISO 13485:2016: 4.2.1, 8.1, 8.2.1, 8.2.6, 8.5
MHLW/PMDA: MO169: 5, 6, 54, 55, 58, 62, 63, 64
MHLW/PMDA: MO169: 37, 43, 54, 55, 58, 60, 61

Japan

Confirm that when the Registered Manufacturing Site plans to make a significant change to a manufacturing processes (e.g. sterilization site change, manufacturing site change), the Registered Manufacturing Site notifies the Marketing Authorization Holder so as the Marketing Authorization Holder can take appropriate regulatory actions [MHLW MO169: 29].

Confirm that the person operating the Registered Manufacturing Site has determined and implemented effective arrangement for communicating with the Japanese Marketing Authorization Holder in relation to customer feedback, including customer complaints, and advisory notices [No.169: 29].

Medical Device Adverse Events and Advisory Notices Reporting
The Medical Device Adverse Events and Advisory Notices Reporting process may be audited as a linkage from the Measurement, Analysis and Improvement process.

Clause and Regulation
ISO: ISO 13485:2016: 4.2.1, 7.2.3, 8.2.2, 8.2.2, 8.2.3, 8.3.3
MHLW MO169: 62.6

Japan

Marketing Authorization Holders are required to implement post market safety activities in accordance with domestic (Japanese) regulatory requirements in addition to the QMS requirements.
The persons operating the Registered Manufacturing Sites are not required to report any adverse event directly to a Regulatory Authority, but shall report any adverse event which meets the criteria specified by the Ordinance for Enforcement of PMD Act Article 228-20.2 to the Marketing Authorization Holder
[MHLW MO169: 62.6].
Verify that the person operating the Registered Manufacturing Site provides events which meets the following criteria defined by the Ordinance for Enforcement of PMD Act Article 228-20.2 (see below), to the Marketing Authorization Holder in a timely manner.
- The following malfunction events which may cause or may have caused health damage:
- Serious event (domestic and foreign)
- Unlabeled non-Serious event (domestic)
- The following Adverse Reaction events which was caused or might have been caused by the malfunction of a medical device:
- Serious event (domestic and foreign)
- Unlabeled non-Serious event (domestic)
- Any action taken for preventing the occurrence or expansion of public health hazard in relation to a medical device which is marketed in foreign countries and is equivalent to the one marketed in Japan. The action includes but not limited to:
- Suspension of manufacturing, importing or selling
- Recall and
- Abolishment.

- Study report that indicates:
- Possibility of event of cancer and other serious illness, injury or death caused by malfunction of a medical device (domestic and foreign), or by infectious disease arising from usage of a device (domestic and foreign)
- Significant occurrence rate change of event etc. caused by malfunction of a medical device (domestic and foreign)
- Significant occurrence rate change of infectious disease caused by usage of a medical device (domestic and foreign)
- The fact that a medical device is less effective than claimed when approved.
Marketing Authorization Holders are required to report advisory notices to Regulatory Authorities
[PMD Act 68-11].
Confirm that the person operating the Registered Manufacturing Site has determined and implemented effective arrangement for communicating with the Marketing Authorization Holder in relation to advisory notices
[MHLW MO169: 29].

Note: Persons operating Registered Manufacturing Sites are not required to report any advisory notice directly to regulatory authority, but shall communicate with the Marketing Authorization Holder, so they can take necessary regulatory actions.

32 • JAHANGIR ASADI

2nd Edition

Design and Development

The purpose of the Design and Development process is to control the design of a medical device and to assure that the device meets user needs, intended use, and its specified requirements. Attention to design and development planning, identifying design inputs, developing design outputs, verifying that design outputs meet design inputs, validating the design, controlling design changes, reviewing design results, transferring the design to production, and compiling the appropriate records will help a medical device organization assure that resulting designs will meet user needs, intended uses, and requirements. Review of the Design and Development process will also provide an opportunity to evaluate how the medical device organization has utilized risk management activities to ensure design inputs are comprehensive and meet user needs, to confirm that risk control measures that were planned have been implemented in the design, and to verify that risk control measures are effective in controlling or reducing risk.

Clause and Regulation
ISO: ISO 13485:2016: 4.1.1, 4.2.1, 7.1, 7.3.10, 7.3.2
MHLW/PMDA: MO169:5, 6, 26, 30, 11, 27, 31

Japan

Class 1 devices are not required to comply with the requirements of MHLW MO169:30-36, which are equivalent to the requirement of design and development in ISO13485 [MHLW MO169:4.1].
For the Marketing Authorization Holder, confirm if the Marketing Authorization Holder has submitted a new application, a change application, or a change notification to PMDA/ a Registered Certification Body, when applicable [PMD Act 23-2-5.1, 23-2-5.11, 23-2-5.12, 23-2-23.1, 23-2-23.6, 23-2-23.7].
For the Registered Manufacturing Site, confirm if the site has a mechanism to communicate with the Marketing Authorization Holder about device modifications, so the Marketing Authorization Holder can take appropriate actions. If a critical medical device modification has happened in the Registered Manufacturing Site, confirm if the Registered Manufacturing Site has communicated with Marketing Authorization Holder about the change [MHLW MO169: 29].

Production and Service Controls

The purpose of the Production and Service Controls process is to manufacture products that meet specifications. Developing processes that are adequate to produce devices that meet specifications, validating (or fully verifying the results of) those processes, and monitoring and controlling those processes are all steps that help assure the result will be devices that meet specified requirements. After completing the audit of the medical device organization's Production and Service Controls process, the audit team will return to the Management process to make a final decision of whether top management ensures that an adequate and effective quality management system has been established and maintained at the medical device organization.

Clause and Regulation
ISO: ISO 13485:2016: 7.1, 7.2.1, 7.5.1, 8.2.5, 8.2.6
MHLW/PMDA: MO169: 6, 24, 25, 26, 27, 40, 41, 45, 53, 54, 57

Japan

The requirements for delivery, installation, and servicing of a particular device should have already been evaluated and addressed by the medical device organization during design and development and planning for product realization.

If risk control measures were identified involving the delivery, installation, and servicing for a particular device, confirm that the necessary processes have been implemented to ensure the risk control measures are in place. For example, a medical device organization may have identified that in order for a medical imaging device to give accurate images, servicing must be performed by trained personnel according to specific instructions.

Risk control measures might include warnings on the imaging device that only authorized personnel should service the device and the design of a unique tool to access the inside of the device that is only provided to authorized service personnel.

Reviewing a validation

During review of a validation study, determine when applicable whether:

- The instruments used to generate the data were properly calibrated and maintained
- Predetermined product and process specifications were established
- Sampling plans used to collect test samples are based on a statistically valid rationale
- Data demonstrates predetermined specifications were met consistently
- Process tolerance limits were challenged
- Process equipment was properly installed, adjusted, and maintained
- Process monitoring instruments were properly calibrated and maintained
- Changes to the validated process were appropriately challenged (if applicable)
- Process operators were appropriately qualified.

Purchasing

The intent of the Purchasing process is to ensure that purchased, sub-contracted, or otherwise received products and services conform to specified requirements. The medical device organization is expected to establish and maintain documented controls for planning and performing purchasing activities. The controls necessary depend on the effect of the product on the quality, safety, and effectiveness of the finished device. Effective purchasing processes incorporate purchasing requirements and specifications, the selection of acceptable suppliers based on the capability of the suppliers to provide acceptable product, the performance of necessary acceptance activities, and maintenance of the required quality records.

The management representative is responsible for ensuring that the requirements of the quality management system have been effectively defined, documented, implemented, and maintained. Prior to the audit of a process, it may be helpful to interview the management representative to obtain an overview of the process and a feel for management's knowledge and understanding of the process.

Clause and Regulation
ISO: ISO: ISO 13485:2016: 4.1.2, 4.1.3, 4.1.5, 7.1, 7.4.1, 7.4.2, 7.4.3

Japan

Planning

In planning product realization, the medical device organization must determine as appropriate the quality objectives and requirements for the purchased products, the processes, documents, and resources specific to the purchased products, the criteria for purchased product acceptance, and the required verification, monitoring, inspection, and test activities specific to the purchased products. Planning of product realization often begins in the design and development of the product, including the translation of the design into production specifications. The translation of the design into production specifications includes the establishment of specified requirements for purchased product.

Quality objectives

Quality objectives are typically expressed as a measurable target or goal. The planning of product realization should include consideration of how the purchased product, the criteria for purchased product acceptance, and the required verification, monitoring, inspection, and test activities specific to the purchased product will achieve the quality objectives.

* Some examples of QOB include:
* Number of complaints -v- number of parts shipped
* On-time delivery %
* Supplier parts rejected
* Comparison of internal audit findings -v- external audit findings
* Achieving a certain accuracy if you're developing product - based software
* Annual Post-market surveillance
* Auditing our system for regulatory compliance

Some managers believe that the reward for hard work should be a paycheck. That's sort of like telling your children that they get to eat for doing something you're proud of. Employees are not children, but you are responsible for developing them into more valuable employees so that they can be promoted. If there is no incentive, your team will not be engaged. Therefore, pick a reward that is proportional to the bottom-line impact. Five percent of the bottom-line impact is what I like to target, but you would be amazed at how effective a few small rewards at each milestone can be. If you have trouble getting management approval for rewards, remind your boss of the bottom-line impact and link the rewards closely to the impact.

Japan

MDSAP
Audit Checklist

		REQUIREMENTS
4 Quality management system		
4.1 General requirements		
		Has the organization:
		a) identified the processes needed for the quality management system and their application throughout the organization (see 1.2)?
		b) determined the sequence and interaction of these processes?
		c) determined criteria and methods needed to ensure that both the operation and control of these processes are effective?
		d) ensured the availability of resources and information necessary to support the operation and monitoring of their processes?
		e) monitored, measured, and analyzed these processes
		f) implemented actions necessary to achieve planned results and maintain the effectiveness of these processes?
		Does the organization manage these processes in accordance with the requirements of this International Standard?
		Where an organization chooses to outsource any process that affects product conformity with requirements, does the organization ensure control over such processes?
		Is the control of such outsourced processes identified within the quality management system? (see 8.5.1)
4.2.1 General		

Doc. Reference	Adequate?	Stage I (clauses marked *)	Stage II
	Y/N	Initials	Initials

		REQUIREMENTS
		Does the quality management system documentation include:
		a) documented statements of a quality policy and quality objectives?
		b) a quality manual?
		c) documented procedures required by this international standard?
		d) documents needed by the organization to ensure the effective planning, operation and control of its processes?
		e) records required by this International Standard (see 4.2.4)?
		f) any other documentation specified by national or regional regulations?
		Has the organization established and maintained a file for each type or model of medical device either containing or identifying documents defining product specifications and quality system requirements (see 4.2.3)?
		Do these documents define the complete manufacturing process and, if applicable, installation and servicing?
	EU	Does the file contain or refer to the location of objective evidence establishing the safety and effectiveness of the device as required by Annex 1 of the MDD? (MDD Annex I)
	4.2.2 Quality manual	
		Has the organization established and maintained a quality manual that includes:
		a) the scope of the quality management system, including details of and justification for any exclusion and/or non-application (see 1.2)?
		b) the documented procedures established for the quality management system, or reference to them?
		c) a description of the interaction between the processes of the quality management system?

Doc. Reference	Adequate?	Stage I (clauses marked *)	Stage II

	REQUIREMENTS
	Does the quality manual outline the structure of the documentation used in the quality management system?
Japan	Confirm that the products distributed in the Japanese market, are approved/ certified/ notified with PMDA/ Registered Certification Bodies [PMD Act: -2-23 ,(1) 5-2-23 1) 12-2-23 ,(1) 23)]. For a manufacturing site which conducts primary design, primary assembly, sterilization, domestic storage until final release of products, confirm that the site is registered by MHLW. [PMD Act: 4-2-23 ,3-2-23]
EU	Are the applicable sections of the Medical Device Directive (MDD) included in the specified requirements throughout the documented quality system? Interpretation: A statement only indicating compliance/conformity with the relevant international or EU regulatory requirements is not acceptable.
4.2.3 Control of documents	
	Are documents required by the quality management system controlled?

Doc. Reference	Adequate?	Stage I (clauses marked *)	Stage II

		REQUIREMENTS
		Is a documented procedure established to define the controls needed:
		a) To review and approve documents for adequacy prior to issue?
		b) To review and update as necessary and re-approve documents?
		c) To ensure that changes and the current revision status of documents are identified?
		d) To ensure that relevant versions of applicable documents are available at points of use?
		e) To ensure the documents remain legible and readily identifiable?
		f) To ensure that documents of external origin are identified and their distribution controlled?
		g) To prevent the unintended use of obsolete documents and to apply suitable identification to them if they are retained for any purpose?
		Does the organization ensure that changes to documents are reviewed and approved either by the original approving function or another designated function which has access to pertinent background information upon which to base its decisions?
		Does the organization define the period for which at least one copy of obsolete controlled documents shall be retained?
		Does this period ensure that documents to which medical devices have been manufactured and tested are available for at least the lifetime of the medical device as defined by the organization, but not less than the retention period of any resulting record (see 4.2.4), or as specified by relevant regulatory requirements?

Doc. Reference	Adequate?	Stage I (clauses marked *)	Stage II

	REQUIREMENTS
Japan	Confirm that Quality Management System documentation and records in relation to a device are retained by the Registered Manufacturing Site for the following periods [MHLW Ministerial Ordinance No.9.3 ,8.4 :169, 68 ,67]: 15 .1 years for "specially designated maintenance control required medical devices" [or one year plus the shelf life for products when the shelf life or the expiry date (hereinafter simply referred to as the «shelf life») plus one year exceeds 15 years] 5 .2 years for the products other than the 'specially designated maintenance control required medical devices' (or one year plus the shelf life for the products of which the shelf life plus one year exceeds 5 years). 5 .3 years for training records and documentation Note: PMD Act 2.8 defines the term "specially designated maintenance control required medical device" as: A medical device designated by the Minister of Health, Labour and Welfare after hearing the opinion of the Pharmaceutical Affairs and Food Sanitation Council as those whose potential risk to the diagnosis, treatment or prevention of disease is significant without proper control since this kind of equipment requires expert knowledge and skill in examination for maintenance and inspection, repair and other management.
4.2.4 Control of quality records	

Doc. Reference	Adequate?	Stage I (clauses marked *)	Stage II

	REQUIREMENTS
	Are records established and maintained to provide evidence of conformity to requirements and of the effective operation of the quality management system?
	Do records remain legible, readily identifiable and retrievable?
	Has a documented procedure been established to define the controls needed for the identification, storage, protection, retrieval, retention time and disposition of records?
	Does the organization retain the records for a period of time at least equivalent to the lifetime of the medical device as defined by the organization, but not less than two years from the date of product release by the organization or as specified by relevant regulatory requirements?
EU	Has the manufacturer retained for a period ending at least five years after the last product has been manufactured, the records listed in Annex II, 6.1 or Annex V, 5.1 or Annex VI, 5.1 (whichever applies)
5 Management responsibility	
5.1 Management commitment	
	Has top management provided evidence of its commitment to the development and implementation of the quality management system and maintaining its effectiveness by:
	a) Communicating to the organization the importance of meeting customer as well as statutory and regulatory requirements?
	b) Establishing the quality policy?
	c) Ensuring that quality objectives are established?
	d) Conducting management reviews?
	e) Ensuring the availability of resources?
5.2 Customer focus	
	Does top management ensure that customer requirements are determined and met (see 7.2.1 and 8.2.1)?

Doc. Reference	Adequate?	Stage I (clauses marked *)	Stage II

	REQUIREMENTS

5.3 Quality policy	
	Does top management ensure that the quality policy
	a) Is appropriate to the purpose of the organization?
	b) Includes a commitment to comply with requirements and to maintain the effectiveness of the quality management system?
	c) Provides a framework for establishing and reviewing quality objectives?
	d) Is communicated and understood within the organization?
	e) Is reviewed for continuing suitability?
5.4 Planning	
5.4.1 Quality objectives	
	Does top management ensure that quality objectives, including those needed to meet requirements for product (see 7.1a), are established at relevant functions and levels within the organization?
	Are quality objectives measurable?
	Are quality objectives consistent with the quality policy?
5.4.2 Quality management system planning	
	Has top management ensured that:
	a) The planning of the quality management system is carried out in order to meet the requirements given in 4.1, as well as the quality objectives?
	b) The integrity of the quality management system is maintained when changes to the quality management system are planned and implemented?
5.5 Responsibility, authority and communication	
5.5.1 Responsibility and authority	

Doc. Reference	Adequate?	Stage I (clauses marked *)	Stage II

	REQUIREMENTS	
	Has top management ensured that responsibilities and authorities were defined, documented and communicated within the organization?	
	Has top management established the interrelation of all personnel who manage, perform and verify work affecting quality, and ensured the independence and authority necessary to perform these tasks?	
5.5.2 Management representative		
	Has top management appointed a member of management who, irrespective of other responsibilities, has responsibility and authority that includes:	
	a) Ensuring that processes needed for the quality management system are established, implemented, and maintained?	
	b) Reporting to top management on the performance of the quality management system and any need for improvement (see 8.5)?	
	c) Ensuring the promotion of awareness of regulatory and customer requirements throughout the organization?	
5.5.3 Internal communication		
	Has top management ensured that appropriate communication processes have been established within the organization and that communication takes place regarding the effectiveness of the quality management system?	
5.6 Management review		
5.6.1 General		
	Does top management review the organization's quality management system, at planned intervals, to ensure its continuing suitability, adequacy and effectiveness?	

Doc. Reference	Adequate?	Stage I (clauses marked *)	Stage II

	REQUIREMENTS
	Does this review include assessing opportunities for improvement and the need for changes to the quality management system, including the quality policy and quality objectives?
	Are records from management reviews maintained (see 4.2.4)?
5.6.2 Review input	
	Does the input to management review include information on:
	a) Results of audits?
	b) Customer feedback?
	c) Process performance and product conformity?
	d) Status of preventive and corrective actions?
	e) Follow-up actions from previous management reviews?
	f) Changes that could affect the quality management system?
	g) Recommendations for improvement?
	h) New or revised regulatory requirements?
5.6.3 Review output	
	Does output from the management review include any decisions and actions related to:
	a) Improvements needed to maintain the effectiveness of the quality management system and its processes?
	b) Improvement of product related to customer requirements?
	c) Resource needs?
6 Resource management	
6.1 Provision of resources	

Doc. Reference	Adequate?	Stage I (clauses marked *)	Stage II

	REQUIREMENTS
	Does the organization determine and provide the resources needed:
	a) To implement the quality management system and to maintain its effectiveness?
	b) To meet regulatory and customer requirements?
6.2 Human resources	
6.2.1 General	
	Are personnel performing work affecting product quality competent on the basis of appropriate education, training, skills and experience?
6.2.2 Competence, awareness and training	
	Does the organization:
	a) determine the necessary competence for personnel performing work affecting product quality?
	b) Provide training or take other actions to satisfy these needs?
	c) Evaluate the effectiveness of actions taken?
	d) Ensure that its personnel are aware of the relevance and importance of their activities and how they contribute to the achievement of the quality objectives?
	e) Maintain appropriate records of education, training, skills and experience (see 4.2.4)?
6.3 Infrastructure	
	Does the organization determine, provide and maintain the infrastructure needed to achieve conformity to product requirements?
	Infrastructure includes, as applicable:
	a) Buildings, workspace and associated utilities
	b) Process equipment, both hardware and software
	c) Supporting services such as transport or communication

Doc. Reference	Adequate?	Stage I (clauses marked *)	Stage II

	REQUIREMENTS	
	Does the organization establish documented requirements for maintenance activities, including their frequency, when such activities or lack thereof can affect product quality?	
	Are records of such maintenance maintained (see 4.2.4)?	
	Has the organization determined and does it manage the work environment needed to achieve conformity to product requirements?	
	a) Has the organization established documented requirements for health, cleanliness and clothing of personnel if contact between such personnel and the product or work environment could adversely affect the quality of the product (see 7.5.1.2.1)?	
	b) If work environment conditions can have an adverse effect on product quality, has organization established documented requirements for the work environment conditions and documented procedures or work instructions to monitor and control these work environment conditions (see 7.5.1.2.1)?	
	c) Does the organization ensure that all personnel who are required to work temporarily under special environmental conditions within the work environment are appropriately trained or supervised by a trained person [see 6.2.2 b)]?	
	d) If appropriate, are special arrangements established and documented for the control of contaminated or potentially contaminated product in order to prevent contamination of other product, the work environment or personnel (see 7.5.3.1)?	
7 Product realization		
7.1 Planning of product realization		
	Has the organization planned and developed the processes needed for product realization?	

Doc. Reference	Adequate?	Stage I (clauses marked *)	Stage II

	REQUIREMENTS
	Is the planning of product realization consistent with the requirements of the other processes of the quality management system (see 4.1)?
	In planning product realization, has the organization determined the following, as appropriate:
	a) Quality objectives and requirements for products?
	b) The need to establish processes, documents, and provide resources specific to the product?
	c) Required verification, validation, monitoring, inspection and test activities specific to the product and the criteria for product acceptance?
	d) Records needed to provide evidence that the realization processes and resulting product meet requirements (see 4.2.4)?
	Is the output of this planning in a form suitable for the organization's method of operations?
	Does the organization establish documented requirements for risk management throughout product realization and are records arising from risk management maintained (see 4.2.4)?
EU	Does the supplier evaluate the need for risk analysis throughout the design process and maintain records of any risk analysis performed? (MDD Annex 1)

7.2.1 Determination of requirements related to the product

Doc. Reference	Adequate?	Stage I (clauses marked *)	Stage II

	REQUIREMENTS
	Has the organization determined:
	a) Requirements specified by the customer, including the requirements for delivery and post-delivery activities?
	b) Requirements not stated by the customer but necessary for specified or intended use, where known?
	c) Statutory and regulatory requirements related to the product?
	d) Any additional requirements determined by the organization?
EU	Vefiy that manufacturing maintains files containing or refer to the location of objective evidence establishing the safety and effectiveness of the device as required by Annex 1 of the MDD. Verify that the manufacturer followed a defined and effective process to establish and maintain a file containing documents defining product specifications and quality system requirements for each newa and existing type/modes of medical devices. Since the last audit, has the manufacturer introduced new products in the EU? Has the manufacturer followed a defined and effective process to obtain an approval from the Notified Body to CE mark a product prior to selling it in the EU? (does not apply to class I devices)

Doc. Reference	Adequate?	Stage I (clauses marked *)	Stage II

	REQUIREMENTS
Japan	Verify that that a «Application for Marketing Approval» or « Notification for Marketing» has been submitted by the MAH; and that the manufacturing facility has been registered. 1) Class 2, class 3, and class 4 medical devices except for the devices specified by the requirement of PMD Act: 223-23 (1): An "Application for Marketing Approval" shall be submitted to PMDA by the Marketing Authorization Holder to receive authorization for marketing a medical device in Japan. [PMD Act: 1) 5-2-23)] An "Application for QMS Audit" shall also be submitted to PMDA by the Marketing Authorization Holder, when they do not have an effective QMS Certificate for the device. [PMD Act: 5-2-23 7) ,(6))] 2) Class 2 and class 3 medical devices which are specified by the requirement of PMD Act: 1) 23-2-23): An "Application for Marketing Certification" shall be submitted to a Registered Certification Body (RCB) by the Marketing Authorization Holder to receive authorization for marketing a medical device in Japan. [PMD Act: 1) 23-2-23)] An "Application for QMS Audit" shall also be submitted to an RCB by the person, when the person does not have a valid QMS Certificate for the device. [PMD Act: 4) ,(3) 23-2-23)]. Facility Registration (Registered Manufacturing Site): A medical device manufacturing site which conducts one of the designated manufacturing processes listed below shall be registered: a) Primary Designing, b) Primary assembly, c) Sterilization, and

7.2.2 Review of requirements related to the product

Doc. Reference	Adequate?	Stage I (clauses marked *)	Stage II

	REQUIREMENTS
	Does the organization review the requirements related to the product?
	Is this review conducted prior to the organization's commitment to supply a product to the customer (e.g. submission of tenders, acceptance of contracts or orders, acceptance of changes to contracts or orders)?
	Does the organization ensure that:
	a) Product requirements are defined and documented?
	b) Contract or order requirements differing from those previously expressed are resolved?
	c) The organization has the ability to meet the defined requirements?
	Are records of the results of the review and actions arising from the review maintained (see 4.2.4)?
	Where the customer provides no documented statement of requirement, are the customer requirements confirmed by the organization before acceptance?
	Where product requirements are changed, does the organization ensure that relevant documents are amended and that relevant personnel are made aware of the changed requirements?
7.2.3 Customer communication	
	Has the organization determined and implemented effective arrangements for communicating with customers in relation to:
	a) Product information?
	b) Enquiries, contracts or order handling, including amendments?
	c) Customer feedback, including customer complaints? (see 8.2.1)
	d) Advisory notices? (see 8.5.1)
7.3 Design and development	

Doc. Reference	Adequate?	Stage I (clauses marked *)	Stage II

	REQUIREMENTS

7.3.1 Design and/or development planning	
	Has the organization established documented procedures for design and development?
	Does the organization plan and control the design and development of product?
	During the design and development planning, does the organization determine:
	a) The design and development stages?
	b) The review, verification, validation and design transfer activities (see Note) that are appropriate at each design and development stage?
	c) The responsibilities and authorities for design and development?
	Does the organization manage the interfaces between different groups involved in design and development to ensure effective communication and clear assignment of responsibility?
	Is planning output documented, and updated as appropriate, as the design and development progresses? (See 4.2.3)
7.3.2 Design and development inputs	
	Have inputs relating to product requirements been determined and records maintained (see 4.2.4)?
	Do these inputs include:
	a) Functional, performance and safety requirements, according to the intended use?
	b) Applicable statutory and regulatory requirements?
	c) Where applicable, information derived from previous similar designs?
	d) Other requirements essential for design and development?
	e) Output(s) of risk management (see 7.1)?

Doc. Reference	Adequate?	Stage I (clauses marked *)	Stage II

	REQUIREMENTS
	Are these inputs reviewed for adequacy and approved?
	Are requirements complete, unambiguous and not in conflict with each other?
7.3.3 Design and development outputs	
	Are the outputs of design and development provided in a form that enables verification against the design and development input, and is it approved prior to release?
	Do design and development outputs:
	a) meet the input requirements for design and development?
	b) Provide appropriate information for purchasing, production and for service provision?
	c) Contain or reference product acceptance criteria?
	d) Specify the characteristics of the product that are essential for its safe and proper use?
	Are records of the design and development outputs maintained (see 4.2.4)?
7.3.4 Design and development review	
	At suitable stages, are systematic reviews of design and development performed in accordance with planned arrangements (see 7.3.1):
	a) To evaluate the ability of the results of design and development to meet requirements?
	b) To identify any problems and propose necessary actions?
	Do participants in such reviews include representatives of functions concerned with the design and development stage(s) being reviewed, as well as other specialist personnel (see 5.5.1 and 6.2.1)?
	Are records of the results of the reviews and any necessary actions maintained (see 4.2.4)?
EU	Does the supplier evaluate the need for risk analysis throughout the design process and maintain records of any risk analysis performed? (MDD Annex 1)

Doc. Reference	Adequate?	Stage I (clauses marked *)	Stage II

	REQUIREMENTS

7.3.5 Design and development verification	
	Is verification performed in accordance with planned arrangements (see 7.3.1) to ensure that the design and development outputs have met the design and development input requirements?
	Are records of the results of the verification and any necessary actions maintained?

7.3.6 Design and development validation	
	Is design and development validation performed in accordance with planned arrangements (see 7.3.1) to ensure that the resulting product is capable of meeting the requirements for the specified application or intended use?
	Is validation completed prior to the delivery or implementation of the product (see Note 1)?
	Are records of the results of validation and any necessary actions maintained (see 4.2.4)?
	As part of design and development validation, does the organization perform clinical evaluations and/or evaluation of performance of the medical device, as required by national or regional regulations (see Note 2)?

7.3.7 Control of design and development changes	
	Are design and development changes identified and records maintained?
	Are changes reviewed, verified, and validated, as appropriate, and approved before implementation?
	Does the review of design and development changes include evaluation of the effect of the changes on constituent parts and product already delivered?
	Are records of the results of the review of changes and any necessary actions maintained?

Doc. Reference	Adequate?	Stage I (clauses marked *)	Stage II

	REQUIREMENTS
Japan	For the Marketing Authorization Holder: When applicable, confirm the Marketing Authorization Holder has submitted a new application, a change application, or a change notification to PMDA/ a Registered Certification Body. For the Registered Manufacturing Site: Confirm the site has a mechanism to communicate with the Marketing Authorization Holder about device modifications so the Marketing Authorization Holder can take appropriate actions when necessary. If a critical medical device modification has occurred at the Registered Manufacturing Site, confirm if the Registered Manufacturing Site has communicated the change to the Marketing Authorization Holder. A change to a medical device which is approved/certified by PMDA/a Registered Certification Body marequire the Marketing Authorization Holder to submit a change application or a change notification [PMDAct ,(1) 5-2-23 23-2-23 ,(6) 23-2-23 ,(1) 23-2-23 ,(12) 5-2-23 ,(11) 5-2-23 7))]. Changes that require a change application or a change notification are those which directly impact the safety and efficacy of thdevice; and/or the intended use, materials, etc. approved during marketing approval / certification. The Registered Manufacturing Site shall communicate changes with the Marketing Authorization Holder when the Registered Manufacturing Site plans such changes. This allows the Marketing AuthorizationHolder to take any necessary regulatory actions mentioned above [MHLW MO29 ;169]. Examples of changes that may require an application or a notification include, but are not limited to: • Design; Composition; Raw material; Sterilization method; • Manufacturing method; Manufacturing site; Patient or user safety features; Operating parameters or conditions for use; Indication for use; Shelf life; Performance specification.

Doc. Reference	Adequate?	Stage I (clauses marked *)	Stage II

	REQUIREMENTS
EU	Do documented procedures identify the need to report essential changes to the Notified Body, (MDD Annex II, V, VI, 3.4)

7.4 Purchasing

7.4.1 Purchasing process

	Has the organization established documented procedures to ensure that purchased product conforms to specified purchase requirements?
	Is the type and extent of control applied to the supplier and the purchased product dependent upon the effect of the purchased product on subsequent product realization or the final product?
	Does the organization evaluate and select suppliers based on their ability to supply product in accordance with the organization's requirements?
	Have criteria for selection, evaluation and re-evaluation been established?
	Are records of the results of evaluation and any necessary actions arising from the evaluation maintained (see 4.2.4)?

Doc. Reference	Adequate?	Stage I (clauses marked *)	Stage II

	REQUIREMENTS
Japan	For Marketing Authorization Holder: If the Marketing Authorization Holder (MAH) has outsourced to a Registered Manufacturing Site (RMS) any process that affects product conformity with requirements, verify the MAH has performed the necessary verification that the RMS has an appropriate quality management system. If the site of a supplier is a Registered Manufacturing Site, verify the MAH has performed the necessary verification that the supplier has an appropriate qualitymanagement system [MHLW MO65 :169].

For Registered Manufacturing Sites: If the RMS has outsourced to another RMS any process that affects product conformity with requirements, confirm the outsourcing RMS has performed the necessary verification that the outsourced RMS has an appropriate quality management system. If the site of a supplier is an RMS, verify the purchase controlling RMS has performed the necessary verification that the supplier has an appropriate quality management system [MHLW MO65 :169]. |
7.4.2 Purchasing information	
	Does purchasing information describe the product to be purchased, including where appropriate:
	a) Requirements for approval of product, procedures, processes and equipment?
	b) Requirements for qualification of personnel?
	c) Quality management system requirements?
	Does the organization ensure the adequacy of specified purchase requirements prior to their communication to the supplier?
	To the extent required for traceability given in 7.5.3.2, does the organization maintain relevant purchasing information, i.e. documents (see 4.2.3) and records (see 4.2.4)?

Doc. Reference	Adequate?	Stage I (clauses marked *)	Stage II

	REQUIREMENTS

7.4.3 Verification of purchased product		
		Has the organization established and implemented the inspection or other activities necessary for ensuring that purchased product meets specified purchase requirements?
		Where the organization or its customer intends to perform verification at the supplier's premises, does the organization state the intended verification arrangements and method of product release in the purchasing information?
		Are records of the verification maintained (see 4.2.4)?
7.5 Production and service provision		
7.5.1 Control of production and service provision		
7.5.1.1 General Requirements		
		Does the organization plan and carry out production and service provision under controlled conditions?
		Do the controlled conditions include, as applicable:
		a) The availability of information that describes the characteristics of the product?
		b) The availability of documented procedures, documented requirements, work instructions, reference materials and reference measurement procedures as necessary?
		c) The use of suitable equipment?
		d) The availability and use of monitoring and measuring devices?
		e) The implementation of monitoring and measurement?
		f) The implementation of release, delivery and post-delivery activities?
		g) The implementation of defined operations for labeling and packaging?

Doc. Reference	Adequate?	Stage I (clauses marked *)	Stage II

	REQUIREMENTS
	Does the organization establish and maintain a record (see 4.2.4) for each batch of medical devices that provides traceability to the extent specified in 7.5.3 and identifies the amount manufactured and amount approved for distribution?
	Is the batch record verified and approved?
7.5.1.2 Control of production and service provision — Specific requiremen	
7.5.1.2.1 Cleanliness of product and contamination control	
	Does the organization establish documented requirements for cleanliness of product if:
	a) Product is cleaned by the organization prior to sterilization and/or its use, or
	b) Product is supplied non-sterile to be subjected to a cleaning process prior to sterilization and/or its use, or
	c) Product is supplied to be used non-sterile and its cleanliness is of significance in use, or
	d) Process agents are to be removed from product during manufacture?
	If product is cleaned in accordance with a) or b) above, the requirements contained in 6.4 a) and 6.4 b) do not apply prior to the cleaning process.
7.5.1.2.2 Installation activities	
	If appropriate, does the organization establish documented requirements which contain acceptance criteria for installing and verifying the installation of the medical device?
	If the agreed customer requirements allow installation to be performed other than by the organization or its authorized agent, does the organization provide documented requirements for installation and verification?
	Are records of installation and verification performed by the organization or its authorized agent maintained (see 4.2.4)?

Doc. Reference	Adequate?	Stage I (clauses marked *)	Stage II

	REQUIREMENTS
7.5.1.2.3 Servicing activities	
	If servicing is a specified requirement, does the organization establish documented procedures, work instructions and reference materials and reference measurement procedures, as necessary, for performing servicing activities and verifying that they meet the specified requirements?
	Are records of servicing activities carried out by the organization maintained (see 4.2.4)?
7.5.1.3 Particular requirements for sterile medical devices	
	Does the organization maintain records of the process parameters for the sterilization process which was used for each sterilization batch (see 4.2.4)?
	Are sterilization records traceable to each production batch of medical devices (see 7.5.1.1)?
7.5.2 Validation of processes for production and service provision	
7.5.2.1 General requirements	
	Does the organization validate any processes for production and service provision where the resulting output cannot be verified by subsequent monitoring or measurement? (this includes any processes where deficiencies become apparent only after the product is in use or the service has been delivered)
	Does validation demonstrate the ability of the processes to achieve planned results?
	Has the organization established arrangements for these processes including, as applicable:
	a) Defined criteria for review and approval of the processes?
	b) Approval of equipment and qualification of personnel?
	c) Use of specific methods and procedures?
	d) Requirements for records (see 4.2.4)?
	e) Re-validation?

Doc. Reference	Adequate?	Stage I (clauses marked *)	Stage II

	REQUIREMENTS
	Has the organization established documented procedures for the validation of the application of computer software (and changes to such software and/or its application) for production and service provision that affect the ability of the product to conform to specified requirements?
	Are such software applications validated prior to initial use?
	Are records of validation maintained (see 4.2.4)?
7.5.2.2 Particular requirements for sterile medical devices	
	Has the organization established documented procedures for the validation of sterilization processes?
	Are sterilization processes validated prior to initial use?
	Are records of validation of each sterilization process maintained (see 4.2.4)?
7.5.3 Identification and traceability	
7.5.3.1 Identification	
	Does the organization identify the product by suitable means throughout product realization and does the organization establish documented procedures for such product identification?
	Has the organization established documented procedures to ensure that medical devices returned to the organization are identified and distinguished from conforming product [see 6.4 d)]?
7.5.3.2 Traceability	
7.5.3.2.1 General	
	Has the organization established documented procedures for traceability?
	Do such procedures define the extent of product traceability and the records required (see 8.3 ,4.2.4 and 8.5)?
	Does the organization control and record the unique identification of the product, where traceability is a requirement (see 4.2.4)?

Doc. Reference	Adequate?	Stage I (clauses marked *)	Stage II

	REQUIREMENTS
EU	Does the manufacturer have procedures identifying the requirements of labeling and instructions for use as defined in MDD, Annex 1 point 13, and is regulations for CE marking included in these procedures. (MDD 3, Article 17 and Annex 12).
	Are language requirements defined in procedures for the information identified in MDD, Annex 1point 13 for the applicable markets.
7.5.3.2.2 Particular requirements for active implantable medical devices and	
	In defining the records required for traceability, does the organization include records of all components, materials and work environment conditions, if these could cause the medical device not to satisfy its specified requirements?
	Does the organization require that its agents or distributors maintain records of the distribution of medical devices to allow traceability and that such records be available for inspection?
	Are records of the name and address of the shipping package consignee maintained (see 4.2.4)?
7.5.3.3 Status identification	
	Does the organization identify the product status with respect to monitoring and measurement requirements?
	Is the identification of product status maintained throughout production, storage, installation and servicing of the product to ensure that only product that has passed the required inspections and tests (or released under an authorized concession) is dispatched, used or installed?
7.5.4 Customer property	
	Does the organization exercise care with customer property while it is under the organization's control or being used by the organization?

Doc. Reference	Adequate?	Stage I (clauses marked *)	Stage II

medical devices

	REQUIREMENTS
	Does the organization identify, verify, protect and safeguard customer property provided for use or incorporation into the product?
	If any customer property is lost, damaged, or otherwise found to be unsuitable for use, is this reported to the customer and are records maintained (see 4.2.4)?
7.5.5 Preservation of product	
	Has the organization established documented procedures or documented work instructions for preserving the conformity of product during internal processing and delivery to the intended destination?
	Does this preservation include identification, handling, packaging, storage and protection, and also apply to the constituent parts of a product?
	Has the organization established documented procedures or documented work instructions for the control of product with a limited shelf-life or requiring special storage conditions?
	Are such special storage conditions controlled and recorded (see 4.2.4)?
7.6 Control of monitoring and measuring devices	
	Does the organization determine monitoring and measuring to be undertaken and the monitoring and measuring devices needed to provide evidence of conformity of product to determined requirements (guide reference 7.2.1)?
	Has the organization established documented procedures to ensure that monitoring and measurement can be carried out and are carried out in a manner that is consistent with the monitoring and measurement requirements?

Doc. Reference	Adequate?	Stage I (clauses marked *)	Stage II

	REQUIREMENTS
	Where necessary to ensure valid results, is measuring equipment:
	a) Calibrated or verified at specified intervals, or prior to use, against measurement standards traceable to international or national measurement standards; where no such standards exist, is the basis used for calibration or verification recorded?
	b) Adjusted or re-adjusted as necessary?
	c) Identified to enable the calibration status to be determined?
	d) Safeguarded from adjustments that would invalidate the measurement result?
	e) Protected from damage and deterioration during handling, maintenance and storage?
	Does the organization assess and record the validity of the previous measuring results when the equipment is found not to conform to requirements?
	Does the organization take appropriate action on the equipment and any product affected?
	Are records of the results of calibration and verification maintained (see 4.2.4)?
	When used in the monitoring and measurement of specified requirements, is the ability of computer software to satisfy the intended application confirmed prior to initial use and reconfirmed as necessary ?
8 Measurement, analysis and improvement	
8.1 General	

Doc. Reference	Adequate?	Stage I (clauses marked *)	Stage II

	REQUIREMENTS
	Does the organization plan and implement the monitoring, measurement, analysis and improvement processes needed:
	a) To demonstrate conformity of the product?
	b) To ensure conformity of the quality management system?
	c) To maintain the effectiveness of the quality management system?
	Does this include determination of applicable methods, including statistical techniques, and the extent of their use?
8.2 Monitoring and measurement	
8.2.1 Feedback	
	As one of the measurements of the performance of the quality management system, does the organization monitor information relating to whether the organization has met customer requirements?
	Have the methods for obtaining and using this information been determined?
	Has the organization established a documented procedure for a feedback system [see 7.2.3 c)] to provide early warning of quality problems and for input into the corrective and preventive action processes (see 8.5.2 and 8.5.3)?
	If national or regional regulations require the organization to gain experience from the post-production phase, does the review of this experience form part of the feedback system (see 8.5.1)?
Japan	Confirm that the personnel operating the Registered Manufacturing Site has determined and implemented effective arrangements for communicating with the Japanese Marketing Authorization Holder in relation to customer feedback, including customer complaints, and advisory notices [MHLW MO29 :169].
8.2.2 Internal audit	

Doc. Reference	Adequate?	Stage I (clauses marked *)	Stage II

	REQUIREMENTS
	Does the organization conduct internal audits at planned intervals to determine whether the quality management system
	a) Conforms to the planned arrangements (see 7.1), to the requirements of this International Standard and to the quality management system requirements established by the organization?
	b) Is effectively implemented and maintained?
	Is an audit programme planned, taking into consideration the status and importance of the processes and areas to be audited, as well as the results of previous audits?
	Are the audit criteria, scope, frequency and methods defined?
	Does selection of auditors and conduct of audits ensure objectivity and impartiality of the audit process (e.g. auditors shall not audit their own work)?
	Are the responsibilities and requirements for planning and conducting audits, and for reporting results and maintaining records (see 4.2.4) defined in a documented procedure?
	Does management responsible for the area being audited ensure that actions are taken without undue delay to eliminate detected nonconformities and their causes?
	Do follow-up activities include the verification of the actions taken and the reporting of verification results? (see 8.5.2)
8.2.3 Measurement and monitoring of processes	
	Does the organization apply suitable methods for monitoring and, where applicable, measurement of the quality management system processes?
	Do these methods demonstrate the ability of the processes to achieve planned results?

Doc. Reference	Adequate?	Stage I (clauses marked *)	Stage II

	REQUIREMENTS
	When planned results are not achieved, is correction and corrective action taken, as appropriate, to ensure conformity of the product?
8.2.4 Monitoring and measurement of product	
8.2.4.1 General requirements	
	Does the organization monitor and measure the characteristics of the product to verify that product requirements have been met?
	Is this carried out at appropriate stages of the product realization process in accordance with the planned arrangements (see 7.1) and documented procedures (see 7.5.1.1)?
	Is evidence of conformity with the acceptance criteria maintained?
	Do records indicate the person(s) authorizing release of the product (see 4.2.4)?
	Does the organization ensure that product release and service delivery do not proceed until the planned arrangements (see 7.1) have been satisfactorily completed?
8.2.4.2 Particular requirement for active implantable medical devices and ir	
	Does the organization record (see 4.2.4) the identity of personnel performing any inspection or testing?
8.3 Control of nonconforming product	
	Does the organization ensure that product which does not conform to product requirements is identified and controlled to prevent its unintended use or delivery?
	Are the controls and related responsibilities and authorities for dealing with nonconforming product defined in a documented procedure?

Doc. Reference	Adequate?	Stage I (clauses marked *)	Stage II

medical devices

	REQUIREMENTS
	Does the organization deal with nonconforming product by one or more of the following ways?
	a) By taking action to eliminate the detected nonconformity
	b) By authorizing its use, release or acceptance under concession
	c) By taking action to preclude its original intended use or application
	Does the organization ensure that nonconforming product is accepted by concession only if regulatory requirements are met?
	Are records of the identity of the person(s) authorizing the concession maintained (see 4.2.4)?
	Are records of the nature of nonconformities and any subsequent actions taken, including concessions obtained maintained (see 4.2.4)?
	When nonconforming product is corrected, is it subject to re-verification to demonstrate conformity to the requirements?
	When nonconforming product is detected after delivery or use has started, does the organization take action appropriate to the effects, or potential effects, of the nonconformity?
	If product needs to be reworked (one or more times), does the organization document the rework process in a work instruction that has undergone the same authorization and approval procedure as the original work instruction?
	Prior to authorization and approval of the work instruction, is a determination of any adverse effect of the rework upon product made and documented (see 4.2.3 and 7.5.1)?
8.4 Analysis of data	

Doc. Reference	Adequate?	Stage I (clauses marked *)	Stage II

		REQUIREMENTS
		Does the organization establish documented procedures to determine, collect and analyse appropriate data to demonstrate the suitability and effectiveness of the quality management system and to evaluate if improvement of the effectiveness of the quality management system can be made?
		Does this include data generated as a result of monitoring and measurement and from other relevant sources?
		Does the analysis of data provide information relating to:
		a) Feedback (see 8.2.1)?
		b) Conformity to product requirements? (See 7.2.1)
		c) Characteristics and trends of processes and products including opportunities for preventive action?
		d) Suppliers?
		Are records of the results of the analysis of data maintained (see 4.2.4)?
8.5 Improvement		
8.5.1 General		
		Does the organization identify and implement any changes necessary to ensure and maintain the continued suitability and effectiveness of the quality management system through the use of the quality policy, quality objectives, audit results, analysis of data, corrective and preventive actions and management review?
		Does the organization establish documented procedures for the issue and implementation of advisory notices and are these procedures capable of being implemented at any time?

Doc. Reference	Adequate?	Stage I (clauses marked *)	Stage II

	REQUIREMENTS
Japan	Confirm that the personnel operating the Registered Manufacturing Site have determined and implemented effective arrangements for communicating with the Marketing Authorization Holder in relation to advisory notices [MHLW MO29 :169]. Note: Personnel operating Registered Manufacturing Sites are not required to report any advisory notice directly to the regulatory authority but shall communicate with the Marketing Authorization Holder, so the MAH can take any necessary regulatory actions.
EU	Are the procedures for Vigilance reporting in conformance with MDD Annex II, V, and VI (MEDDEV 1-2.12)
	Are records of all customer complaint investigations maintained (see 4.2.4)?
	If investigation determines that the activities outside the organization contributed to the customer complaint, is relevant information exchanged between the organizations involved (see 4.1)?
	If any customer complaint is not followed by corrective and/or preventive action, is the reason authorized (see 5.5.1) and recorded (see 4.2.4)?
	If national or regional regulations require notification of adverse events that meet specific reporting criteria, does the organization establish documented procedures to such notification to regulatory authorities?
Japan	Verify that the person operating the Registered Manufacturing Site provides events which meet the criteria defined by the Ordinance for Enforcement of PMD Act Article 2) 20-228) to the MarketingAuthorization Holder in a timely manner.

Doc. Reference	Adequate?	Stage I (clauses marked *)	Stage II

	REQUIREMENTS
EU	Are procedures for the reporting of recall to the relevant competent authority and the NB compliant? (MDD, Annex II, V, VI, 3.1)
8.5.2 Corrective action	
	Does the organization take action to eliminate the cause of nonconformities in order to prevent recurrence and are corrective actions appropriate to the effects of the nonconformities encountered?
	Has a documented procedure been established to define requirements for:
	a) Reviewing nonconformities (including customer complaints)?
	b) Determining the causes of nonconformities?
	c) Evaluating the need for action to ensure that nonconformities do no recur?
	d) Determining and implementing action needed, including, if appropriate, updating documentation (see 4.2)?
	e) Recording of the results of any investigation and of action taken (see 4.2.4)?
	f) Reviewing the corrective action taken and its effectiveness?
8.5.3 Preventive action	
	Does the organization determine action to eliminate the causes of potential nonconformities in order to prevent their occurrence and are preventive actions appropriate to the effects of the potential problems?

Doc. Reference	Adequate?	Stage I (clauses marked *)	Stage II

	REQUIREMENTS
	Has a documented procedure been established to define requirements for:
	a) Determining potential nonconformities and their causes?
	b) Evaluating the need for action to prevent occurrence of nonconformities?
	c) Determining and implementing action needed?
	d) Recording of the results of any investigations and of action taken (see 4.2.4)?
	e) Reviewing preventive action taken and its effectiveness?

Doc. Reference	Adequate?	Stage I (clauses marked *)	Stage II

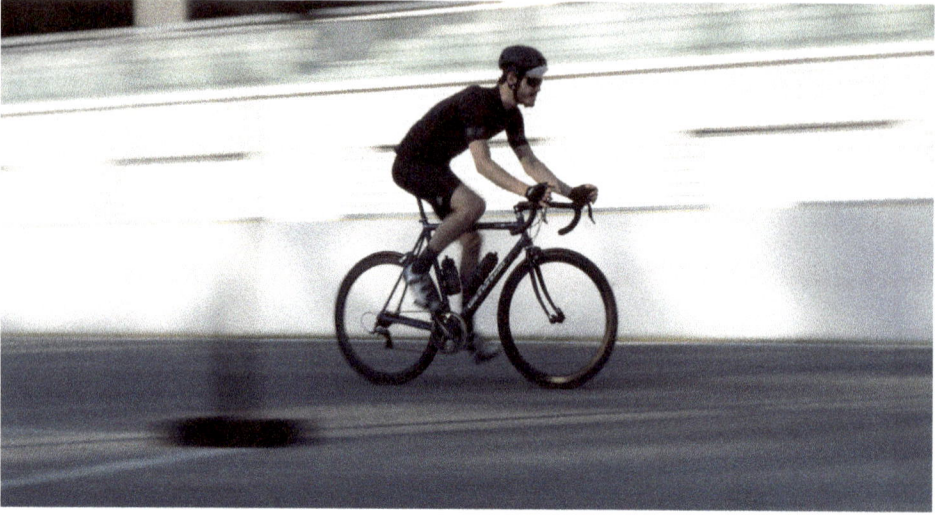

The system is working for you (the system is fully integrated along your processes and eases your operations).

You are working for the system
(the system is beside your operations and looks as an
additional burden.)

Advice for manufacturers planning certification
Firstly, you should confirm that the device(s) your company manufactures can be defined as a medical device under ISO 13485 standards; or, if you provide a medical device service, that your service is related to a product defined as a medical device. Getting ISO 13485 certification is challenging and requires commitment so, secondly, it's important that your leadership team confirms that holding the certification will add value to your company, meet its business objectives and support its strategy. While holding the full certification is not strictly necessary, as your company can still conform to and benefit from ISO 13485 standards without being externally certified, it does clearly demonstrate to all stakeholders that you comply with its requirements.

If you do want to become independently certified there are two phases; the first covers documentation, while the second implements your quality management system and audits it. You must carry out phase two within six months of completing phase one.

ISO 13485 certification costs
For companies who wish to be fully ISO 13485 certified, there are associated costs for external, independent certification. Although you may be under cost pressure, it's important to work with an independent auditor who will add real value to your company during the certification process. In this highly regulated industry, choose a reputable auditing company with extensive expertise rather than one that enables you to gain certification at the lowest price.

BIBLIOGRAPHY

Bibliography:

Astrini, N. (2018). ISO 9001 and performance: a method review. Total Quality Management & Business Excellence, doi: 10.1080/14783363.2018.1524293.

Asadi,J, Easy ISo 13485:2016, Silosa Consulting Group, 2022

Bou-Llusar, J. C., Escrig-Tena, A. B., Roca-Puig, V., & Beltra´n-Martı´n, I. (2005). To what extent do enablers explain results in the EFQM excellence model? International Journal of Quality & Reliability Management, 22(44), 337-353.

Chatzoglou, P., Chatzoudes, D., & Kipraios, N. (2015). The impact of ISO 9000 certification on firms' financial performance. International Journal of Operations and Production Management, 35(1), 145-174. https://doi.org/10.1108/IJOPM-07-2012-0387

Definition of the terms "medical device" and "in vitro diagnostic (IVD) medical device". Global Harmonization Task Force;

Guidelines for regulatory auditing of quality systems of medical device manufacturers – Part 1: general requirements

Global Medical Devices Nomenclature System (GMDN) [website] (https://www. gmdnagency.org, accessed 2 February 2017).

FDA website address: fda.gov

Gigante, N., & Ziantoni, S. (2015). L'edizione 2015 della norma ISO 9001, 2015. Retrieved from:https://www.accredia.it/app/uploads/2015/12/6050_5_L__700_edizione_2015_della_norma_ISO_9001___Arch__Gigante__Dr__Ziantoni.pdf

ISO (2015a). ISO 9001 - Quality management systems – requirements. Geneva: International Organization for Standardization.

Role of standards in the assessment of medical devices. Global Harmonization Task Force; 2008 ISO (2018). ISO 19011 - Guidelines for auditing management systems quality management systems. Geneva: International Organization for Standardization.

ISO (2019). ISO 9000 Family - Quality Management. Retrieved from: https://www.iso.org/home.html.

Wilson, J. P., & Campbell, L. (2018). ISO 9001:2015: the evolution and convergence of quality management and knowledge management for competitive advantage. Total Quality Management and Business Excellence, pp. 1-16. https://doi.org/10.1080/ 14783363.2018.1445965

ONLINE
EDUCATION

START YOUR ONLINE COURSE NOW AFTER YOU HAVE COMPLETED READING THIS BOOK, DO YOUR QUIZZES AND RECEIVE YOUR

INTERNATIONAL TRAINING CERTIFICATE OF :

ISO 13485
MDSAP

JOIN US AT:

www.Silosa.ca

	MDSAP **Vol.1** AUSTRALIA
	MDSAP **Vol.2** Brazil
	MDSAP **Vol.3** Canada
	MDSAP **Vol.4** Japan
	MDSAP **Vol.5** USA

www.ingramcontent.com/pod-product-compliance
Lightning Source LLC
Chambersburg PA
CBHW040756220326
41597CB00029BB/4960